Tashanda Mosley

Walking

in

Newness

Fight, Faith, Freedom

In Loving Memory of

Mrs. Callie Mae McCoy-Mosley

March 1, 1926 - February 17, 2018

#CallieStrong

Walking in Newness: Fight, Faith, Freedom

Dedication

To Pastor Ruben and Linda Lewis, and my GOBC
family.

Had I not walked through those doors in 2016, I may
have never been brought to life. The way the love of
Christ works through this place is beyond explanation.
It must be seen, never heard about. It cannot be put into
words. Here, I have learned to accept that I am deeply
loved and there is absolutely nothing anyone can do
about it. Here, I have been taught radical faith and bold
worship. The type of faith you cannot see with the
human eye or understand with a logical mental state,
but you know it to be true because it is so. Because He is
so. The type of worship that pulls at you until you're
bellowing out words of praise and on your knees crying
tears of joy and submission. When the transformation is
placed so strongly on you, your previous life becomes
distorted images. You, Grace, I will never forget where I
was brought to my knees and forced to cry out for help. I
will never forget, after years of falsities, I have
encountered the ability to decipher what Love truly is
and that it remains still.

To Daddy, Mama, Will Jr., Michelle, Cedric, Shelia, Timothy, and Wanda.

Far from perfect, but you are all perfectly mine. I am who I am because of you. You make me stronger. You'll never know how much motivation you instill in me. You'll never know the importance of your presence in my life. And even through the bickering, nothing, no one, no devil in hell could ever come against what we have.

To my spiritual sisters -

The best part of you all is your fiery faith and diligence. The second-best part is none of you require or expect a dedication because it truly is your love for Yahweh that keeps you focused on His will for your lives and others. To ask for fellow prayer warriors, and to be provided with you instantaneously, I could never disregard your roles in my life. I don't have to mention names. I'll only have to mention that I love you dearly, and I'm more than happy to war with you any day!

And finally, to Love.

The funny this is You don't require many words because You speak boldly for You. But in the same breath, there will never be enough words to explain your presence. You broke me down. You pulled me apart, limb by limb. You took my heart and held it up in Your hands and You breathe life. You removed the bullets. You removed the broken glass. You urged me to endure the pain. You cleansed me and stitched my wounds with my tears and Your Blood. You stood me to my feet, even as it felt of sizzling shards of broken glass. Then You spoke. "Now, live." And I did. Not only did I live, I survived.

Only because You broke me and Loved me back together.

Walking in Newness: Fight, Faith, Freedom

Before...

"December 30, 2015

So, this is life... It's less than two days before year 2016, and I'm here nurturing my nothing but worthless life. I thought after years of remaining faithful and hopeful, doing good things and being a good person, that maybe I'd have something to show for it. Instead here I am, at nothing. I have a job, in which I'm thankful for. I can pay my bills and put food on the table. I am also in my second and final year of graduate school, which I'm extremely thankful for as well. I have been able to master something I thought I would never get to, maintaining As and Bs for the last year and a half. It's been strenuous and stressful, but it's been worth the pain and wait. I wouldn't give it up for the world.

Then there's the rest of my life... I'm still single. Not the worst thing in the world, of course. I've definitely experienced worse, but I think it's the "side effects" of being single. For instance, the feeling of wanting to settle when you know you deserve better or maybe you don't. Or maybe I just don't! Having to "tone down" who you are because he may not like that side of you. Having everyone and everything remind you that you're single and lonely. Reminding you that no one wants you, or that you're not allowed to have companionship or to be in love. Yes, it sucks. Bad!!

Yet, this brings me to the next part of my worthless life... I try to bring light and love to every single person I encounter. See, I know that it can brighten your day just from someone being kind towards you. I don't do it because of obligation. I do it because I think everyone should know he/she is being thought about. So, just as I feel that everyone deserves to be cared for and thought of, I want the same thing for me, but I couldn't feel any less than love. At this point in my life, I think all people want from me is what I can do for them. Counsel; Listen; You know, do the things that they want me to do. I've been so disregarded in these past two years that it has become habitual for me. I'm simply just numb to it. It's so easy for people to hurt me but it's so easy for me to forgive. I truly believed I was in the thoughts of no one. I'm over 300 pounds but no one sees me until I'm benefiting them. No one hears me until I'm encouraging and uplifting them. No one loves me! I think family "love" me because it's more of an automatic obligation, but how many truly care for me? None if you ask me! This isn't just me feeling sorry for myself. This isn't just a pity party. I feel alone with no one to lean on. No one to understand me. No one to ease the pain. At this point, I've lost all motivation to be anything more than I am now. A minimum wage working fat woman, with too many losses and failures to give anything else another shot. I've given my all to people and I've still come up short.

I may not have had many boyfriends, but I've felt so much pain in just this year alone that it's starting to feel right. Even worst, all this is coming from people who claimed that they love me or care for me.

Someone that said I meant something to them. I think people really expect me to never feel. I think they think that I'm that person that is okay with being the afterthought. My cousin always says she's the afterthought, but I don't think that's the case for her. I think people always think about her, but her intimidating mannerism makes it hard for people to come to her first or directly. I, on the other hand, am always the afterthought. I have a twin sister, same face and everything, and people love her. They call her. They text her. They want to be around her. Me? I'm kind of forced to be happy with whatever makes everyone else happy.

I've had lots of thoughts of suicide lately. Running out in front of a car, or just cutting myself. Maybe it'll ease the pain. Maybe there's some relief. I don't know really, but I do know when I'm dead and gone they'll think of me then. They'll say great things about me. They'll love me or maybe they won't!"

This is dedicated to the young man or young woman whom the enemy has tricked into believe he/she is alone. That there is no hope for them. That they should just end it. This is what fear looks like. Not fear on my part, but fear of the enemy. His final attempt, his final strategy; because even he knew God was about to pick me up the turn my life around. He had to try to get me to cancel my own life. It would be the only way. Poetic; His only way to get me.

This was life before God. Life before I realized just how significantly loved I am by the Father. Just how treasured I am. Just how much I am worth. Just how much more others were praying for me. Just how powerful the Spirit of Christ is inside of me.

This is proof that God can and will absolutely and completely transform your life!

Walking in Newness: Fight, Faith, Freedom

PRELUDE

March 27, 2016. Easter Sunday.

The day I died and came to life in the very same second.

When most people think of Easter Sunday, we imagine little girls in their pretty floral and lace dresses, or little boys dressed handsomely in a creased shirt and pants, completed with a bowtie. Young men looking all dapper in a three piece with freshly cut hair, and young ladies with newly purchased and overly expensive chiffon dresses and hats big enough to provide shade for one fifth of the church. Your appointed religious leader ministering to the congregation about the crucifixion of Jesus Christ and how this marvelous Being rose on the third day, having taken on the tremendous burden of the world's sins.

A supernatural Rebirth.

It's ironic, isn't it? The same Sunday observed to celebrate Jesus Christ's death and resurrection, verifying Himself as the Son of God, was the same day God pulled me from death. Nope, not that ironic, at all. More like strategic. He had set me up. Now I am in no way close to being the Son of God. However, God chose to adopt us into sonship through Jesus Christ. Therefore, I am His and He has the right to do with me as He pleases, including bringing me back to life.

This is what my soul experienced the day I hesitantly walked into the faithful doors of Grace Outreach Bible Church in Greenville, Mississippi, pastored by Ruben and Linda Lewis. Now the first thing you will never be able to deny about this place of worship is the powerful presence of Yahweh. You're supposed to sense it when you stride into any building of worship because that's it intended purpose, but of twenty-eight years, I had never felt that emotion until this very day. There's a calming, welcoming feeling that comes over you. However, in the same moment, there's something in you that wants to move. That wants to know more about this feeling you're undergoing. This is what I first experienced. I guess looking back, it was God's way of picking me off the tree, checking for my ripeness, removing me from a former life of depression, seclusion, and unhappiness by bringing me to a life of clarity, love, joy, faith, and most importantly; living a comfortably uncomfortable life lead by the power of the Holy Spirit.

I believe the most important thing to understand before proceeding is nothing about trusting God says "easy." Nothing about trusting His will says comfort, and nothing about your journey of faith will be relaxed. While Yahweh will take away your burdens and give you your heart desires, it will be a battle to turn from our earthly wants and needs to His. It's like making the choice to jump off a cliff, hoping there will be someone to catch you at the bottom. When we make the decision to give our life *back* to Him; we are signing an agreement that states we are willing to go through the turmoil to get to back to Him, to experience His love, to know Him, and ultimately giving Him absolute control of your life.

Let me clarify. We are always His. We don't have to *do* to be loved by Him. We're already loved, even throughout our flaws, transgressions, disrespect, rebellion, and disobedience. He will not put burden on you because you go astray. It only seems like a burden because of the fight between the flesh and the Holy Spirit. I like to say its protection. He knows you more than you do, and He fights the enemy even as you don't see the attacks. The struggles come from you turning from your wicked ways because the enemy will persecute you. The enemy will deprecate you. The enemy will taunt you.

I know you were expecting me to give you a list of foods and exercises, and maybe even quick fixes to this whole weight loss thing like lose 20 pounds in two weeks by drinking lemon and cayenne pepper water for fast results. This is not one of those cases! It's actually the complete opposite. This is losing fifty pounds in three months and being at a standstill for the next six months. This is working two jobs and taking on stressful workloads, therefore having no time to work out. This is dealing with demons from your past that you thought you'd gotten rid of. This is real life. Everything that can happen will happen. This is truly a journey of faith and trust. Discipline and patience were seemingly two of my worst enemies. Only because I had yet to understand that I was the only individual preventing myself from moving into a life of greatness. I thought I needed someone to push me. I thought I needed someone to care. I thought I needed someone to pick up the pieces. That's great and all and kudos to those great supporters out there but coming into a life of newness is not accomplished with new people, new surroundings, and new opportunities; it begins with a new way of thinking. How you see yourself has everything to do with the outcomes of *every* situation you encounter and living the life the Father sees you is the only way to alter that contaminated mode of thinking. Every opportunity, every relationship, and every failure will be shaken by Him!

So, no, this is not about weight loss. This is about me and my experiences with Yahweh. This is about you being fed up with failing yourself. This is about His open door-policy with you. This is about fight, faith, and freedom!

Tashanda Mosley

How Did I Get Here?

I guess there is no better place to start than from the beginning. My earliest memory of having to battle with being overweight and depression: my childhood. I know, I know. It's so cliché, but I truly have been overweight as long I could remember. In elementary school, I remember always being larger than most of my classmates. I remember always being conscious of my size. Hoping I wasn't in anyone's space or making sure my stomach didn't touch the backs of the other children as I was shifting through the isle. It was a very embarrassing thought as a child in second and third grade, even if no one knew I was thinking it.

Growing up, my mother was the breadwinner. She brought home the bacon. It may have been the scraps and fat leftover after the pig had been robbed of all the good stuff. She brought it home nevertheless, and it had gotten us through the longest days and toughest nights. My mother only had an eighth-grade education. She left her parents' house at the sweet age of sixteen and never went back. She moved to the big city of Greenville and found a job working as a waitress at Morrison Café, which most Greenvillians remember as Picadilly's. She eventually went on to obtain her G.E.D. and start cosmetology school. However, upon finishing and preparing for the state board, she went into labor and gave birth to my brother.

On the other hand, my father graduated high school in which he proceeded on to obtain his associates in HVAC. He completed two years at Mississippi Valley State University. However, he did not complete his degree. My mom likes to say we got our smarts from my dad, and I must admit the man was brilliant when it came to the books. He was very knowledgeable in his field and people trusted his work. After several unfortunate events took place in his life, he retired from the workforce.

Unfortunately, with so much idol time on his hands, he picked up a nasty habit of drinking.

Let's be clear, I will not blame him for this habit. This is a man that has always worked, knew the value of a dollar, and was a successful business man at one point. When he had an accident at work and it forced him into disability, he felt useless. There is a mental burden of not being able to provide for your family that will take a complete toll on any good man. This isn't the only reason he picked up on drinking though. There were other reasons that it could have been prevented, but I will not bash my father. It's the past. We'll let that be.

Well since we're talking about how I got here, we'll have to talk about his part too right?

I truly felt like my father did not love me. He never showed any type of affection. Never told me he was proud of me. I was never a daddy's girl. If anything, he degraded me. Time after time, he would come in drunk and sit my brother, sister, and

I down, and would lecture about us about God knows what for hours. Somehow, "mother wit" ended up every conversation. For those of you who don't know, "mother wit" is basically common sense. Trust me, I know. I was kind of forced to know. He used to always say, *"If you don't stand for something, you'll fall for anything."* He wanted us to challenge him because he knew he intimidated us. Yes, I was afraid of my father. He scared me.

My mother, on the other hand, had to kind of make up where my father lacked. She had to make sure we were comfortable. He wasn't a very good provider after he stopped working and turned to alcohol. We could only afford to get the inexpensive but unhealthy foods like junk food and fast foods; foods that caused diabetes, high blood pressure, high cholesterol, heart diseases, and obesity. These same foods became comfort for me. Well honestly, there was never comfort, but it hid my problems for a little while. My mom always made sure we had plenty of comfort. We certainly didn't always have it all. As a matter of fact, we struggled tons, but as a child with no cares or no worries, you never really notice the struggle. All you know is your parents have food on the table, clothes on your back, and a roof over your head. Not once do you consider what they had to go through to get and keep the necessities.

That's not to say that we went didn't have to go without some things. A lot of times we didn't have what our peers had. We didn't have the financial privileges that many children could. When we got money, it often went to the house. I don't ever remember my siblings and me complaining to my parents about unnecessary expenses and desires or being ungrateful for the things they provided. Even though as children we didn't have real responsibilities, we were definitely aware of our household income situation. With only one working parent and a father that battled alcoholism, it was usually easy to give up on money to benefit the household as a whole.

If it was ever anything we had to sacrifice, my mother made sure we had *something* to eat. It may not always have been exactly what we wanted, but we had something to consume before we closed our eyes for bed at night.

As a matter of fact, when she obtained extra money, she tended to over feed us. I believe it was because often times we didn't have much money, so to compensate she wanted to make sure we didn't starve. The overfeeding became a habit of hers. Because she was mama, we did as we were told. Also, since we struggled, we appreciated the food we had.

As a child, I didn't see anything wrong with this. I only saw a parent trying to feed his/her children by making sure their hunger was satisfied when they closed their eyes at night. Little did we all know though, it caused a repetitive habit. A habit that wasn't evident until I was well in my teenage years.

Walking in Newness: Fight, Faith, Freedom

2

Me, Myself, and the Hovering

For as long as I can remember, I always felt... followed. Ha. Creepy right? It might make sense to some of you, others not so much, but as much "loneliness" as I experienced during my childhood and adolescent years, there was always some sort lingering over me. Often times, emerging from grade school ages, I questioned why was I created? I was almost shocked that I was living and breathing, and that people physically saw me. I didn't know what I was supposed to do or how long of a time I had to do it. I wanted answers. At that age however, I didn't hear anything or maybe I was too young to *hear* the voice of God.

I recall like it was yesterday one particular incident that I knew God had or would set me apart from my close peers and family members. As stated before, the enemy attacked me early with the feeling of loneliness. At a certain time period at twelve or thirteen, I had grown overly emotional; the spirit of depression tried to overtake me. I will still cry at the drop of a hat now, but mostly in worship and in awe of Our Father. During this time the loneliness had set in heavily. It was my first time wondering what my family members' lives would be like without my presence. With a notebook in front of me, I laid on my bedroom floor. I cannot recall whether I was doing homework or simply writing, but I do remember feeling so alone and so incompetent; like I just did not belong, period. My twin sister was there too. And suddenly, I'm crying. At this moment my sister ran to get my mom. The poor child didn't know what had hit her sister. My mom came in and inquired about the tears. I honestly could not give her a straight answer, or maybe I should say I didn't know how to answer without her thinking I had lost my mind. The feeling was nearly unbearable, and I wanted to scream out. I wanted to yell at wherever this feeling was that made me feel so lost and without. But I couldn't tell my mom this. I didn't want her to judge me.

I guess I should have gone ahead and told her because she still thought I'd lost my mind for laying on the bedroom crying for no apparent reason. I remember her saying I was going to send myself into a nervous breakdown and that she was going to send me to a counselor. It only made me cry harder. At that moment, I wanted a counselor - thinking maybe they could tell me just what in God's name was going on with me.

This wasn't the last of me feeling like this. It happened much more throughout high school. However, I did learn to keep it to myself to avoid the mocking and being misunderstood.

I also found another outlet: The opposite sex.

Of course, when puberty starts, girls get boy crazy and vice versa. However, it wasn't so much the boys that captivated me. It was the attention. And yes, as young girls we do seek attention from the boys. But the enemy programmed me to believe that I needed this attention, that this attention was going to be necessary for me to live; that if there was ever a risk of me losing him, I would have to give in to whatever he wanted from me or find another one to fill the void and give me that attention I had become dependent on.

But as much as I longed for a man's attention, I never gave in to sexual intercourse in high school. I used to say it was the fear of my mother that prevented me from sexual activity in high school. She told my sister and me that if we got pregnant, we "better put salt and pepper on it and eat!"

No, I was not raised a cannibal. She never put us on contraceptives and she never ever encouraged us to use them. So what my mother meant was don't have sex. If you got pregnant under that roof, you better have some place to go because you couldn't bring it there. Some of you may (or may not) find this a bit harsh. But already having three children trying to make ends meet, the last thing she needed was another mouth to feed. And it never made any sense for a baby to raise a baby. So many of your parents may have other tactics to prevent unprotected sex and teen pregnancy, but this was my mother's and it worked! However, as stated, it was not my mother that kept me from no sex in high school. It was two things.

First: my father via the enemy. Too many times, my sister and I heard that all we would be good for was to lay on our backs and have a house full of children. At the time I was never told how beautiful and significant I am. If I even looked like I had the right answer to the solution, the devil would shoot me down and "remind" me that I "didn't know everything" but to "challenge" him anyway. And he used my father for all of this. I have said once before, but let me reiterate, I do not blame my father for anything anymore. I thank God for the deliverance of that spirit because I realize it was the enemy and not him. My father loves me, and I love him, period.

But you can just about imagine what a young girl such as myself was going through - so naïve and ignorant of the evil spirits and wicked powers that was using my father as their messenger. All I knew at that time was that I was looking at the face of my father, telling me I was nothing and that he didn't care. But the devil knew this. If he could get the first man in my life that was supposed to love me, care for me, and be my first hero, to deny me - then he would set me out on a lifelong quest in search of something I didn't know that I already had. And he knew that nothing would ever satisfy me completely because I would always look to be accepted and loved.

So how did this become my reason to not have sex as a teenager? I simply wanted to prove him wrong. I wanted to show him that I was not some sex crazed teen. I wanted to prove that I could graduate without kids. I wanted to prove to my father that I was not what he said I was. And ultimately, I wanted to make him proud. I wouldn't say it was because I didn't have urges to have sex. I mean come on! But proving him wrong meant everything at the time. This is also where performing came about. If I could prove to him that I was good, maybe he would finally love me or at least accept me.

It didn't dawn on me until later down my road of life, and I do mean much later, that it wasn't my father I was performing for, but the devil. And he never had intentions on loving me, no matter how many times I excelled in a performance.

As a matter of fact, it only made him hate me more, which brings me to my second reason for keeping my virginity intact throughout high school.

Second reason: The Hovering, the presence I could never quite get rid of. While it is pretty obvious that the enemy started with me early, that presence refused to let me go. We frequently attended church, even if my parents couldn't make it. Every Sunday morning, we walked two blocks, with a quarter or two fisted tightly in our hand and listened to The Word.

But even still, I can't say that it was completely church, or maybe this particular church, that brought the hovering. First of all, the hovering was always there; surely before the struggles of obesity and depression, but *especially* during my struggles with obesity and depression.

When I felt like I was in a room full of people and no one saw me, when I cried myself into a deep slumber for whatever reason - there was always a *"but I'm here with you"* feeling. There was a protection. Times where the devil threatened my life, the hovering intensified. At the time, the hovering was not enough to satisfy my flesh. Nevertheless, it was enough to keep me going and apparently, *I* was enough to keep coming back to every day as much as I rejected it.

I guess I should probably explain to you when I started to take notice of Its presence. It was August of 2006. By this time, my faith had a foundation. I had established that I believed in Jesus Christ and the word of God. Even if I didn't always go by the Bible, you couldn't argue with my belief. I knew there had to be some type of purpose to my life, even if I didn't know what it was. I had transferred to community college in Raymond, Mississippi. It was my first time ever being away from family, including my twin sister. And boy, did I cry. At this time, the attacks of loneliness happened frequently, and I had started to accept it, even though I never fully got used to it. *I was never supposed to.* I remember my cousin having some of his friends set my room up and after they left, the tears fell. And they fell, and they fell. Sheesh, I felt so alone.

When I finally got myself halfway together, I was introduced to more people my cousin knew and they kind of took me under their wings; but only because I was his cousin. However, I appreciated their warm welcome. I had like $45 to get grocery and washing detergent. After that $45 was spent, I had no idea where I'd get extra money for anything. Keep in mind, finances still weren't completely up to part in my household, and the last thing I wanted to do was bug my mother about money. She was already doing the best she could, and it was my idea to move on campus.

So, I bought what I could buy and tried not to worry about anything else if it came about. By the end of the month there, the housing department was in search of a new resident's assistant. My cousin was already a resident's assistant, so he put in a good word for me with the housing department director and I got the job. This got me a $1900 scholarship grant, free room and board, with my own room and bathroom. So, now I had a job. But the money wasn't going to be available for a while, so I was still sort of buried with emotions.

One night at work, I was confiding in one of my co-workers about the stress I was under, and she was really being as supportive as any college student could be. It was also her first time away from home and she barely knew how to separate her colored laundry from her whites. She could literally only offer me a listening ear.

In the middle of our conversation, the housing director walked in with a box of washing detergent and a container of bleach. She said my cousin told her that I needed to wash so she brought some over. I was thankful and elated. That was one less thing I had to worry about. I noticed the detergent box was open and something told me to take a look inside.

There, inside a box full of powdery detergent, was a one-hundred-dollar bill.

My mouth dropped opened. I looked up at my co-worker. Her mouth was just as wide as mine. I looked at my housing director like she had clean lost her mind. This woman did not know me. She had only met me once, when she offered me the job. She didn't know anything of my background. I didn't even go through training for the position. I had not set down for lunch with her, or anything. Nothing. She knew nothing about me. And she had just given me washing detergent, bleach, and $100.

Literally, "*Thank you,*" was the only thing I could say, over and over again, tears streaming down my pie face. And she was so humble about it. She acted as if she had not done anything.

When I called home and told my mom about it, she was just as shocked. She said we would have to pay her back for what she did for me. But she wanted to thank her for her kindness. So some days later, I had my cousin's phone, and our housing director came over again. I called my mom and let her speak to her. My mom proceeded to thank her and let her know she would pay her back.

You know what this woman said?

"Pay me for what? I didn't do anything."

My mouth flew open again. Was I hearing her correctly?

She then says, *"You owe me nothing. I only gave her washing detergent."*

Now let me connect to my Southern roots for just a second: Y'ALL... this threw me a loop.

Not only had this woman given me a job, gave me washing detergent and bleach to wash my clothes, $100, but she said she didn't do anything. And guess what? She never ever brought it up again. I have long ago lost contact with this woman, but I will forever be grateful for her generosity.

So, I guess you're saying by now "What does this have to do with the Hovering?" EVERYTHING.

The Hovering, *my* Hovering, my Holy Covering went into protection mode when separated from what I knew. I was only at that community college for a semester. But I truly believe I was directed there for just that semester, on purpose. I believe He needed me to know that He would protect me and that He had every intention of taking exquisite care of me. I'm convinced that Yahweh needed me separate from the comfort zone, the known, so that I could know that He would be present also in the unknown.

Now from this point on, you'll notice me saying *my* Holy Covering instead of the Holy Covering, because I want to establish, that He is mine, and I am His, and He would say the same. His Word promises that He could do exceedingly and abundantly above all that we could ask for or think! But before I could even think it, it is done. He provided, using a complete stranger as a vessel. He went against the school employment procedure, where resident assistants were normally required to do one month of training before the school started to prepare for the upcoming school year and dormitory rules; and he employed me with a job without training or a resume. My remaining time at the school, I wanted for nothing. Things would just fall in my lap. I literally have no idea where the money came from, but it was always there. *Always.*

It was also around this time I started to experience waking up in the wee hours; 3 am to be exact. There was this movie that came out about a young lady that was having exorcisms performed on her. Then, it was probably by the far the scariest thing I had watched, because people had been saying it was based on a true story. It was so scary that I didn't even watch the entire movie. But what I did see had effects on me mentally. I had really gotten in my head that the devil could harm me and there was no hope for me. I remember sometimes when I woke up, I used to see demon faces and I'd be up the remainder of the night, afraid.

The enemy attacked with fear at this time. He helped me create a little cute shell and politely pushed me into it and convinced me that he had nailed the door shut. I was convinced that my comfort zone would keep me safe. Maybe if I stuck to what I knew—the food, the boys, the aggressive behavior—that maybe he would let up off me. But even my comfort didn't keep me safe because the attacks kept coming. I had forgotten just that quickly that the devil would always hate me, and if I gave him just a little wiggle room, his attacks would continue, especially to prevent me from getting to the Most High.

At some point, when fear didn't work, I found prayer to be an option. Well if I can be honest, it might have just been a last resort. (Yes, I was one of Yahweh's hard-headed children.) I don't believe this came to me coincidently. I was definitely led to praying by my Holy Covering. I found that when I prayed or read His Word during these early mornings that there was much peace; sleep found me sooner. Unfortunately, fear had altered my mindset and it wasn't quite as easy to overcome the damage the enemy had done.

But two things of the infinite things to remember about our Holy Covering: He is exceedingly tenacious, and He always wins. While those demons fought against me, they fought for a reason. I may have allowed them to come in, but the enemy also knew what they were fighting against and that in the right moment, the perfect moment, He would snatch me back to His covering in an instant.

However, I do believe Yahweh allowed much of the attacks to go on for many reasons. Remember the story of Job? God gave Satan permission to punish Job, even as he as was an upright servant. God believed and was confident that Job would not curse Him, but Satan spoke otherwise. Now I don't believe God did this to entertain the devil. However, I do believe God wanted to test Job's trust. It's easy to say, *"I love and trust you, God,"* when everything is going well. But what about when it seems the opposite? Yes, praise and rejoice and brag about Him when you and everyone else can see the outpouring of His blessings. But delight in Him even more when the road gets rough and tough, when your circumstances seem to be attacking you all at once. Will you trust Him then?

This is where the real test of love comes. I don't think Yahweh expects trust to come easy. But I do believe He still expects it to come! He also expects you to lean on Him for strength. And this is what I believe God chose to do with me, even in my early years, like Job and all of us. Will I remain faithful? Will I still praise and rejoice? Will I finally cry out to Him?

So, now I see and truly believe many of my attacks were a test of faith and beckoning call, as well. My Holy Covering meant business and He meant to protect me and love me. But to stay protected, I had to be under His covering, and to be under His covering, I needed to answer His call.

Tashanda Mosley

3

One Naïve Little Girl

I know we briefly touched basis on me and the opposite sex earlier. But my pass connection with other men also played a key role in my weight gain and as well how I viewed myself and God as well. As I stated before, my Holy Covering was very protective of me. So not only did He intensify with the side effects of obesity, but also when I was in the presence of the opposite sex. Not just any person of the opposite sex, but the one that gave me the unhealthy attention I desired, and I would give it back. And I guess you'd probably say what's wrong with giving the attention back. Well, in this case, it's a lot wrong with it.

First, because I didn't really *want* to give him the type of attention he was looking for. The attention I was giving was out of my character. The attention I was giving was performance based. *"If I give him this, then he will keep giving me this."* It was very conditional, but I'd fix my mind to keep pushing for it. Secondly, it didn't sit right with my Holy Covering. Even before I knew what the Hovering was exactly, we couldn't help but sort of be in sync because it was always present. So, when I did something that didn't align with my spirit, my Holy Covering didn't hesitate to let me know.

The even crazier thing about this whole thing is I was terrified of boys in school. I didn't want to end up pregnant and I certainly didn't want to physically experience the pain of my first time. I'd heard plenty of stories, and the way my mind was set up then, I had a very low tolerance for pain.

But being the attention seeking, naive girl that I was, I ignored these realities. Yes, I kept pressing the buttons that had the sign written in a black permanent marker that said, *"Do not touch."* And each time I did, I pushed myself further in the mud with each unnecessary (and many times) sexual compliment - boosting egos that need not be boosted.

This type of attention seeking often got me into situations, relationships, and "situation-ships" that wasn't as easy to get out of as it was to get in. Why? Yes, I was a virgin indeed, but I was what men called a "tease." As I had gotten older, I developed the ability to pick up on what young men my age liked, which was sex or something pretty close to it. But since I wasn't having sex, I learned the art of pretending, and I became pretty convincing. And I was able to use my virginity as bait. Knowing a woman was untouched drives a man crazy, and of course I had the upper hand.

You see how the enemy will use the most innocent thing? My body was always meant to glorify God. My virginity was sacred, precious, priceless; and meant to be allowed access only to my husband. But using my desire for the attention against me, I dangled my untouched body in front of men, knowing I never had intentions on giving myself to them. You play that game with a sexually frustrated man one too many times, BOOM, just like that you're liable to have your purity stolen from you or worse, meet an early death.

There was only one time in high school where I came close to *intentionally* losing my virginity. There were many times it could have happened, but this was the only time I probably would have done it. It was my first love. Let's just call him Dee. Dee and I had met when I was about twelve or thirteen. He was initially my cousin's boyfriend (different story, different book!). But we ended up dating throughout my entire time in high school. He was my everything and he knew it. He knew exactly what buttons to push and how to say what he needed to say. I would have done anything for him. I was literally wrapped around his fingers. He gave me the unwholesome attention I so desperately desired. When I had to be at school the next day, we stayed on the phone until 6 in the morning, went to school, and came right back home, just to get on the phone with him and do the same thing over again, as if we hadn't talked in months. Dee is the reason why I desire meaningful conversation. I despise small talk with the opposite sex. Our talks range from religion, sex, family, sex, school, sex, marriage, sex, life goals, and sex. Our conversations were very mature for fifteen and sixteen-year-olds.

Dee knew I was virgin, and yes, he pressured me, heavily. He was not a virgin, but he wanted to be my first. He wanted me to want him to be my first. He wanted me to need him. And you want to know why he could want what he wanted, and I let him? Because he was the first man to tell me he loved me. My father had said it to me once or twice, but at the time I needed it the most, I no longer heard him say it.

So, Dee was that guy. I now believe that because we were both young, Dee never intended to harm me. He made me feel beautiful. He never disrespected me. Never once called me out of my name, always honored my presence, even if there were other girls in his life to keep him "company."

Yes, because I didn't have sex with him, this allowed the opportunity for other women to come in to entertain him. He never admitted to these women. Even now, if I was to call him up and ask if he had other girls while we were together, he'd proudly deny it. But a boy as mature as Dee does not learn what he learned simply from school books. The guy was experienced in life. He had a hard life, and he taught me all he could, including sex if I had let him. But even with the extra entertainment, I was "the girlfriend" and he upheld his boyfriend duties, for the most part.

Dee was the first break up where I know God gave me the strength to perform. We had broken up before, on and off throughout high school. But shortly before I graduated from high school, we experienced a number of misunderstandings and arguments that ultimately led to the breakup.

I still remember the break-up. We'd gotten in an argument and he hung up on me. I think some part of me was just fed up. I called him back and told him that I didn't want to be with him anymore. He said "*Okay,*" and hung up on me again. Later that day, he called back and apologized and said that we should get back together. I told him no and that this was the end of us as a couple. We've actually remained really good friends. But the relationship never rekindled, no matter how many opportunities were presented.

So, by now, you're probably wondering about "*the one.*" Ha, well he came along while I was with Dee. Let's call him D2. I actually developed a little crush on him while Dee and I dated. This brought problems for Dee and I *and* family, but different story. D2 and I didn't officially begin our little "romance" until my sophomore year of college. But before that, we were the best of friends. Honestly, I would have called him anything, just so he could stay in my life. The connection to this man was strangely powerful, especially for a girl that already had a boyfriend. But I also know this is when I started to compare myself to other women and when I tried to conform to what I thought he wanted me to look like. He used to say, *"You're so pretty for a big girl..."* Ugh. If you've ever struggled with obesity and dating, you know what that feeling is like. Basically saying, *"You're cute but not small enough."*

So literally every woman I passed, I would compare myself to her and feel defeated when I summed up that she could take him away from me, even though he was never mine. But he stuck around, dated other women, and flirted with me when it was convenient.

During sophomore year of college, after not speaking for a period of time, he finally made his move. We planned to hang out during Christmas break and those plans stuck. We got together late on Christmas night and chilled in his car. It was somewhat like old times, except now my virginity was at stake. If I thought I was ready to give my all to Dee, I was practically sure I would give it to D2. Because he was my best friend. I'd always wanted to be best friends with my boyfriend. Dee and I were also best friends but the attraction to one another came before the friendship. With D2, our friendship was allowed to grow before the fake romance came. D2 and I shared so much. My mom liked him, and his mom liked me. I was good friends with his siblings. They literally became my second family. We had that "Brown Sugar" kind of friendship. Remember that movie? Yep, that was me and D2.

D2 was also there when my family lost our home due to financial hardships. My mom had lost her job and my dad no longer worked. Things basically plundered, and we were homeless for a short period during my high school senior year.

During this time period, we stayed in two hotels for about a month. And while my boyfriend had no idea about this, D2 knew all about it. And he was there with me through it all, his family included. So, his presence became significant.

After being friends since high school sophomores, we shared our first kiss on Christmas night 2006. I may as well have handed my body over to him right then because at this point I was hooked. I wanted to be with him and not just sexually. I'm talking about walking down the aisle, sixteen bride-maids and groomsmen, moving to Atlanta, starting my career as a registered nurse, and having about eight babies with this man. Crazy, right? Well this was me. He was my *strong* stronghold.

We continued this little thing for nearly three years. Why do I say "thing?" Because it was never a relationship. Ever. No matter how hard I tried to convince myself that it was going somewhere. It just wasn't. So, I tried to force it. How? Well I came up with the *marvelous, bright* idea (I wish you could hear the sarcasm in my voice) that if I had sex with him, he'd finally feel what I feel. Sex was the only thing missing anyways, right? Wrong times seven!

The problem with this is that he always wanted to be my friend. Now every blue moon, he'd give me false hope of the future, but he really wanted to be friends. And he had expressed this several times. But also, God caused his heart to harden towards me too many times to count. Why? So, *I* could walk away. God fought hard for me and I couldn't even see it. But once I made my mind up that he would be my first, there was no convincing me otherwise.

The end of June or early part of July of 2009, I had a dream about the number 7. Everything in this dream surrounded the number 7, and the number 7 seemed to flash in and out the dream.

Now, the obsessed, naïve me thought it was about D2, mainly because there was song that played in the end of the dream that we both loved. This definitely meant we were meant to be, right? Wrong times seven again!

But again, I ran with it. I literally began planning the moment I'd give up virginity to him. I asked D2 what would happen between us once it happened. His response: We'd still be good friends.

God had given me my final warning.

On July 31, 2009, I lost my virginity to D2. And yep, you guessed it. Everything had practically remained the same. Only one other difference had occurred. Those same feelings I expected him to receive had gotten to me. So there I was, stuck with double the feelings and emotions than what I had before; and he'd move on with his life.

Don't think I didn't try again. I was a determined little rugrat! I tried to force a reconnection with D2 and me. I relocated unexpectedly to the same city he resided in at the time. It definitely was not planned but I most certainly was not against it.

After numerous attempts, God gave me another dream. In this dream, I was following D2, trying to get him to *see* me and *hear* me. The walkway became icy and slippery for me, while he walked along completely fine. He walked into a house and I made my way behind him into the house. When I walked into the house, there was complete darkness.

Crystal clear, right?

All of this led to seven years of trying to forgive him, forgiving myself, and facing the holds the enemy had over me.

The number seven plays an extremely significant role in my transformation journey, and this case isn't any different. As a matter of fact, it's the first of the many significance moments with seven. While I thought it meant good, God used the number seven as a warning in the dream. God was trying to caution me that when I give myself to this man, I'd be punished seven years for my disobedience. This punishment would include men that I desired hardening their hearts towards me, shutting down any type of relationship or romance, and seven hard years of singleness, filled with trials and tribulation. And most importantly, I would not be allowed to be in another relationship until I repented and recognized Him, Father Yahweh, as my one true love.

And He meant just that. Because He always keeps His Word.

Walking in Newness: Fight, Faith, Freedom

4

The Setting of Your Mind:

What You Think You Say

Many times, during the writing of this book, I fasted; a lot. Normally when I tried to fast (in my own strength), the most difficult part was usually bearing the aromas pouring from the kitchen. Foods you normally wouldn't find enticing suddenly seem like your last meal on earth; it becomes the apple of your eye. It becomes your next breath. However, in this case, during my recent fasts, the absolute most difficult part is my mental state. And it has absolutely nothing to do with food. Okay, maybe a little. But it's mostly my mind going in constant circles. It's the battle of knowing and understanding the good and the evil. Knowing the voice of Yahweh and being able to decipher when the enemy is trying to come against what God is bringing to me.

Around the end of February and early March of 2017, I began to get too relaxed with the weight loss. Because I was losing the weight in good timing, I allowed myself to make excuses on what I could eat. I rewarded myself for making the progress I'd already made, having no regard to how careless and reckless I was being with body. Completely forgetting that overeating and emotional eating was why I was chosen to make the lifestyle change in the first place.

Each week, I said I'd get back on track. But each passing week, I'd make another excuse and continue down the old path to being bonded to obesity again and allowing food to be my comfort. What others ate, I ate-- fast food and all. I still maintained some of my new eating habits, but I had gotten comfortable again, forgetting that Yahweh makes you *uncomfortable* to purge and transform you.

This wasn't the first time I had gone through this period. Back in 2016, when I initially started the weight loss journey, I lost over 50 lbs between May 1 and mid-July. After that, I somewhat made myself an experiment, thinking that it was the exercising that was more helpful than what I ate. So, I sort of ate what I wanted to, not fully trusting God, but what social media said. By this, I mean I found all types of fad diets that I thought would work because it appeared to have worked for others. And I don't mean to bash others weight loss journey and their chosen paths. But when I heard the Holy Spirit say, *"Just make a few adjustments,"* and I accepted that, I then made Yahweh my official coach. All athletes know that when you don't take note of the information the coach is feeding you, regardless of how great of a player you are, your career will flop when you can't take criticism and correction.

Why do you think the enemy attacks the mind? Because before you say it, you think it. Most of the time you imagine things in your mind first before you actually see them. Truth be told, it's one of your strongest weapons. But if not used properly, it can turn into your worst enemy, *by the enemy.*

Have you ever been called "big-headed?" If you've been called this before or have called someone else this, more than likely the person that's being referred to is viewed as being overly confident. They may get full of themselves and feel unstoppable. Most of the time, this cockiness is already instilled in this person's mind, and it's highly probable that this mentality was instilled in him/her before any sort of results took place.

But it's not about being conceited or arrogant. It's about how your mind is set up. We all don't operate the same way because we all don't have the same conductor.

With the devil behind the wheel, he does one of two things: 1) He makes you that overly confident person that fools you into believing that you can't be touched and that you're the secret behind your own success. You develop this "it's all about me" attitude or "I got mine, you get yours" mentality. 2) He cripples you. He degrades you. You're made to feel defeated and incompetent. He speaks *death* to you. Every inch of hope, energy, and fight is pulled out of you when the devil is allowed to control your mind.

Both of these can be equally as damaging. The devil's intent is to lead you to destruction. But for that "big-headed" person, the ending may hit harder. Why? Because the higher you go, the harder the fall. Keep in mind: the enemy hates you. The only love he has is to see that you are destroyed. He sets you up for failure. So, don't get elevation confused with God's blessings. If you're not exalting *Him*, serving *His* people, and contributing to the building of *His* kingdom, it's likely the devil has his greedy hands on your mind.

Now, with Yahweh directing the show, our Father takes His precious time, and I do mean precious time, with our minds. He loves to love on us. He wants you to know you're the most important thing to Him, because *you are*! He wants you to know He will move heaven and earth for you, because *He* will! He wants you know that He sent His only Son to die especially for you, because *He* did! He wants you to know, acknowledge, and accept the gifts He's given you because *you are gifted*! And He intends to spend your every waking and sleeping moment reminding you.

But funny thing. Like the enemy, God will set you up. He will set you up for a SET UP. He'll set it up all up for you, prepare your miracle, open up positions, make a place for you, and let you just live it up in His glory. But you have to trust Him enough to allow Him to your mind.

Doubt

I remember waking up early one morning, around 5 a.m., getting ready for work. I showered, got dressed, and was out the door by 5:30, trying to get to work at a decent time. Once there, I got to work, moving around hastily trying to finish the duty that I had been assigned to. But I noticed a difference in the way I walked. Every single time I passed a mirror, I was urged to slow down, and look at myself.

However, I wouldn't let myself. I was so wrapped up in work, trying to finish up. Finally getting off some hours later, on my way home, I heard the Holy Spirit say, *"Stop and look at my handiwork."* So, I got home, went into my room to change. Now currently at this time, I had not one but two large mirrors in my room. I watched myself as I put on a new sweater that fitted well at the time of purchase. Now the sweater that fit at the time I bought it, it was almost too big.

I suddenly broke down because I had finally gotten it. *"Stop and look at my handiwork."* It had only been God. Not I. When I stopped operating in my own willpower and strength, and used His, when I least expected it, He transformed my body in His hands, the way He wanted it, taking His time, molding me and shaping me, strategically and carefully. His word says, *"For we are God's*

handiwork, created in Christ to do good works,
which God prepared in advance for us to do."
(Ephesians 2:10, New International Version)

Before 2016, I had made numerous attempts
to lose the weight. Honestly. I was always aware of
my weight and was never completely comfortable. I
always felt like it was more out there for me. Like
losing the weight was always supposed to be a part
of my journey, back to who I was. Back to Christ.
Back to Yahweh.

But the enemy convinced me, made me
believe that I had to have another person to do this
with. I believed that I needed someone to push me. I
remember trying to force my doctor to put me on a
diet, so I wouldn't have to do it myself. He only
suggested it but he never enforced it. I told people
all the time that if I was going to lose weight, they
would have to stay on me. They would have to push
me. I needed to be pushed and I could not do it
alone. This also goes back to needing other's

reassurance and depending on others to validate me.

I tried, time after time with other people, mostly family members. Started but never finished. Never successfully completed goals I mapped out for myself. I think the most I lost when I worked with other people was maybe 20 to 25 lbs. Then I got comfortable, fell back into old habits, gained that weight and more back. It was horrible.

When I failed, I doubted myself. I forced myself to believe that I couldn't take on this journey alone. I had no commitment to the struggle. I doubted the Hovering that had proved Himself constantly to me, over and over again. I doubted Yahweh. I didn't know that the doubt was pushing me into fear. And again, this goes back to the enemy trying to hold my mind captive, because if only I had gotten a glimpse of what Yahweh was about to do in my life, I would have fought him off long ago.

Before I go any further, get this: Doubt cannot exist with the Holy Spirit. It cannot reside in the same place as Christ. You cannot take doubt with you into a journey led by the Holy Spirit; you will never start it because fear and doubt will consume you before you get your foot out of the door. Doubt is impossible's best cousin and nothing about God is impossible.

When God brings you into recollection of who you are to Him, He intends to purge you, doubt included. Why? *"Because the one who doubts is like a wave of the sea, blown and tossed by the wind... such a person is double minded and unstable"* (James 1:6-8, New International Version). Doubt and faith never existed peacefully together. Think about it: You put God and the devil in the same room, and it *will* be war. Literally, one will outweigh the other and the decision of who you allow in relies solely on you. But here's some free information: God does not accept double-mindedness, because it means you can't be trusted with the inheritance and promises He has for you. You can't be a reliable soldier to help build up His kingdom. This is why when you surrender to Him, He purges you *first*, to rid you of any spirit that is not of Him.

And what happens if you chose the devil? Well let's remember he already hates you. You can just about figure out what you can expect from him: more doubt, more deception, more failure, no life.

But God said I was *His* handiwork and that *He* prepared me in advance, meaning that He took pride in me *as* He created me, and no one was about to take the credit for what He had already done in me.

So, I chose God.

Discipline

I remember the *final* time I tried to lose weight with a group of people. It was summer 2015, still in graduate school and at this point, really searching for something, trying to find out who I truly was. My cousin returned from the military and somehow convinced me that he could help me lose the weight. To me this was perfect: ex-military soldier who knew all about pushing and pulling, being assertive, and knew what it was to be physically fit. They fought in war after war, right? Their bodies were built for this. Of course, he knew how to get the weight off. Exactly what I needed. To be pushed.

We struck out - him, two other cousins, and myself, to become healthier than ever. To be an *exercise machine*... (again, you should really hear how my voice reeks of sarcasm).

This may have lasted a good month. Okay, I'll give it six weeks. But after week six or so, I had decided I did not like someone forcing me. I didn't like to be pushed. I didn't like working out in groups. I didn't like discipline.

There. I said it.

It's bad to say, but truth be told, I hated to be disciplined, especially by someone a few months younger than me. Nope, it was not for me. Now don't get me wrong. This same cousin introduced two of my favorite exercises to me: boxing and running. I never saw myself running. Ever. But he pushed me. He helped me to step outside of that comfort zone, into wobbly grounds. When I restarted this lifestyle change the right way, those were the two things I elapsed back to and still are to this day.

It wasn't that I didn't desire to be healthier because I truly did. It was the sticking to it once I'd gotten started it. It was the long wait before results. It was the anxiety and the former mindset I held. Could I really do it? Did I really have to work hard to get these results or was it any way possible for an easy way out?

Truth is there will always be an easier option. But proceed with caution. The easy way means you could stay inside your comfort zone, but God desires to move us outside of that comfort zone. The comfort zone is what brought this food addiction. The comfort zone says it's okay to stay in unhealthy relationships. The comfort zone says you can continue to live in sin and not take responsibility for the actions and consequences. We can't stay there. We have to go.

This is what many of us fail to see: Our minds are not aligned with the Holy Covering. Our faith is not established. Our trust in Him is weak. But this journey? This cannot be done without Him. How many more failed attempts will you have to have before you surrender to His will? What more damage does your body have to suffer through before you take heed to the red flags? How many more lies does the devil have to tell you before you see that disparaging path diminishes your spirit?

Why Not You?

Many times, I asked My Father, *"Why did you choose me for this?"* Many times, you will ask Him, *"Why am I the one for this?"* This is a question I have asked before many times and this is a question that you'll likely find yourself asking quite frequently. From the beginning, I've asked in moments of frustration, when I'm ready to give up, when I thought I had nothing left. Those are the times He just sits back and let me pout and looks down at me with His arms folded, like *"Are you done yet?"*

I recall a perfect example. I was driving to work, and it had already been a very trying day and an even harder day prior. I believe I had a misunderstanding with a family member; arguments with family were always harder on me emotionally. I was just absolutely frustrated. Then on top of being frustrated, I was forced to be patient with waiting. Waiting for the calling that I knew was inevitable. The calling I knew was mine but couldn't have, because I failed to see that I was not ready for it yet. I was just angry. And I was angry with Yahweh. And I asked Him, *"Why did you choose me for this? Why me?"* I told him I didn't want it. I said *"Take it. Please just take it! It's too much!"* I mean I was balling, face wet as the Pacific Ocean.

This wasn't the only time something like this occurred. I had more than several dramatic breakdowns. I could not understand for the life of me why He had chosen me for these tasks. After being obese majority of my life, He chose me to choose a healthier lifestyle and to lose weight. After being an extremely emotional being for 29 years, He chose me to counsel my peers. After seven years of celibacy and six years of singleness, He wanted me to use my singleness as a platform to encourage and inspire others. After revealing to me that I was being prepared to be a wife, He expected me to be patient and wait longer for a mate. What is that? That's Our Father, that's what.

There were many times, I'd gotten upset with Him and would call Him out on it.

Until finally after another breakdown and peace had settled in, my inner witness said, *"Nothing has changed."*

He saw me crying. Saw the hurt I was experiencing. Saw my frustration. And He empathized, never leaving my side.

But He also never changed His mind.

So, I ask Him, *"Why did you choose me for this? What made you stamp my name on it and say, 'This one right here is for Shanda?'"*

Well, He responded through my Pastor, who referenced from 1 Corinthians 1:26-31:

> Brothers and sisters think of what you were when you were called. Not many of you were wise by human standards; not many were influential; not many were of noble birth. But God chose the foolish things of

the world to shame the wise; God chose the weak things of the world to shame the strong. God chose the lowly things of this world and the despised things and the things that are not to nullify the things that are, so that no one may boast before him. It is because of him that you are in Christ Jesus, who has become for us wisdom from God that is, our righteousness, holiness and redemption. Therefore, as it is written: "Let the one who boasts boast in the Lord" (NIV).

Therefore, it's simple really: Because I am weak. Because I have failed. Because my body type made the odds against me. Because they don't expect me to be greater. Because they didn't expect the type of transformation He planned for me. Because without Him, I am nothing. Because I can never truthfully say it was me. Because it's not about me, but about Him. Because He *will* have His glory.

Tashanda Mosley

5

His Temple

As I've continued this journey, I realized that I had to ask God what He desired me to eat. The weight loss isn't always consistent. Many times, I stayed at the same weight for weeks at a time. I believe this is for several reasons: 1) As the weight loss persists, it's important for me to understand that my weight loss journey is not like other, mainly because I was chosen to take a more spiritual route to weight loss. It was not self-initiated. It was not through surgery (no offense to those who have). It was not because I got tired of being overweight, although it played a significant role. No, as tired as I had gotten of being morbidly obese and being extremely uncomfortable with my body, truth is food was my go-to. I *love* to eat. I love great food. I come from a family of self-proclaimed chefs. It's only one true, certified chef in my family and I have the privilege of calling her my twin sister. But I have that family with auntie and cousins, especially my cousin-sister Jackie, that will get in the kitchen and get you right. Get your stomach nice and tight! So, it's very easy to fall captive to food because truth is, it was my comfort. When happy, eat. When upset, eat. When confused, eat. When tired, eat and go to sleep. It wasn't until well after the weight loss journey began when I realized how addicted I was. I believe God chose to show me this because food had become something I depended on rather than depending on Him for my strength. When something hinders your progressive relationship with God, it has to be exposed so the Father can handle that battle for you, which brings me to my next reason. 2) Yahweh is our Source. He's our supplier, our deliverer, our protector, our strength. If we cannot find comfort in Him, we cannot find comfort any place else. Also, if we cannot acknowledge who He is and *how much* He paid for us, we cannot expect prosperity to fall upon us as it would if we did acknowledge Him. I believe God wanted to show me that my body is His body. Jesus Christ is His body, and when He died on the cross, and rose again, we became one with Him. Therefore, He lives in us. So not only is Christ His, but we are His. And because we are His, when you confess, surrender, and began to live a righteous life for Him, He's not going to allow things from the former life to come in and taint your newness, including poor, unhealthy eating habits and choices.

Back in summer 2015, when I started to work out with my cousins, I went to the doctor's office for a check-up and to see about a pulled muscle. Honestly, I just wanted my nurse practitioner to tell me that I couldn't work out for a couple days because of the pulled muscle.

The appointment was normal for the most part, just sort of confirmed for me what I already knew. I had polycystic ovarian/ovary syndrome better known as PCOS. With PCOS, your hormones are imbalanced, and your ovaries are enlarged and their filled with cysts. PCOS' symptoms include abnormal or absence of menstruation, obesity, severe acne, unwanted facial hair, higher risk of being infertile, and even depression.

I'd done research in my late teens, early twenties to find out why I'd suddenly stop having periods at 15. The first doctor led me to believe that it was normal and that I'd just have trouble having children. So, I just lived with it.

But as I got older, the symptoms showed more--the excess unwanted hair, continuous absence of periods, morbid obesity, and depression. You can only imagine what this does to a woman, whose confidence is already shot. I didn't feel like a woman at all.

At the doctor's office, she confirmed what I'd suspected. Her treatment option: birth control. I'd always hated birth control. I had the best birth control already. But she strongly recommended that I take progesterone for 10 days. After, my period would come on and then after that, I was to continue with the birth control until... But if my period didn't start, don't take the birth control.

This wasn't the first time a doctor suggested progesterone and birth control. The progesterone worked but I didn't go back for the birth control. This time around, I took the progesterone for 10 days and had planned to go on with the birth control, just for the sake of having a menstrual period. After the ten days, nothing happened. I waited and waited. Still nothing.

She also said I had a vitamin D deficiency. She suggested yet another pill, a vitamin D pill that would cost me $50-$60 each month. She said I was insulin resistance, which is another part of PCOS that caused skin tags and dark patches. I don't remember her suggesting anything for this.

So now I have a decision to make. Do I just accept this diagnosis, or do I do something about it? Well, God made the decision for me, when He led me to do one of my research papers on polycystic ovarian/ovary syndrome while in graduate school. I gathered up as much as information as possible. Basically, there's not a medical cure. To get a handle on the disorder and the symptoms: lose weight and maintain an active lifestyle.

This was so very strategic of God. The same summer I admitted my dislike for discipline to working out was the same summer He showed me that working out was the only way to rid myself of this thing. Of course, I rebelled and used my pulled muscle as a crutch.

It was also around this time where my depression strengthened. This was probably the worst of the depression spirit ever. Suicide was much more probable at this time than loved ones ever knew. Daily, I walked around my parents, siblings, and other family members and no one knew that I struggled with thoughts of taking my life. Ironically, this was around a period where people felt the need to remind me that I was "too emotional" and that I should probably "tone down my words", and my personal favorite, I was too "wordy."

Obviously, I'm a very wordy person, otherwise I wouldn't be writing this book. But words? Words are one of my passions. I love to write. I love poetry. I love the meanings that words can hold. That's why meaningful conversations are so very important to me. So basically, telling me not to express myself was a hard hit. If I couldn't express myself, what else did I have? The outcome? I shut down. And when I shut down, the devil went in. And God was not having it!

When the medication failed, and my pulled muscle excuse could longer hold, and the depression weighed in, it was like God was began saying, "*Now are you going to trust me*?" At this point, my hands were tied. God was telling me that He was all I had, and with Him I could have everything.

This body that I have and this body that you have are not given to you by accident. It was given to you on purpose *in* purpose. It is meant to birth purpose, and this mandate was given by a purposeful Father. Do you think He carelessly gave you your body? No; your creation, your mind, your gifts, and your body were carefully thought out with strong purpose.

Everything His hands create is meant to glorify Jesus Christ and to build His kingdom, your body included. This body and your body are His temple. The spirit of Christ lives in us. We are one with Him. His word recites, *"Do you not know that your bodies are members of Christ himself? ...But whoever is united with the Lord is one with him in spirit"* (1 Corinthians 6:15, 17, New International Version).

Yes, Christ lives within us. What we put in our bodies affects the spirit that resides there. Notice, when something enters your body that should not be there, your body rejects it or there is some sort of negative impact. Don't believe me: Too much sugar? You get hyped up then you crash. Too much pork? First, a headache then eventually high blood pressure. Sex before marriage? Yes, it feels so good at the time of intercourse. Maybe you even believe that it's an act of your love and affection towards your significant other at first; but then you're reminded that you don't even *like* the person. After a while, you don't understand why you can't let go when the relationship has clearly seen its death.

I guess some readers my say "*Well diabetes run in my family.*" No, our families have *claimed* diseases for generations and no one has chosen to fight against it. But that stops here with you.

How do you think a perfect God creates your body to be defeated? How is a perfect creation made to be filled with diseases? Yes, we battle, and we struggle but we have *always* been made to overcome, because the One who overcame death resides purposely inside of us. And if He can take a beating, carry a cross, be nailed to that cross, and then rise on the third day, surely, He knows full well how to tend to the temple that we use daily.

The doctors told me I needed a manmade medication to do something a woman's body was naturally created to do. God said use my body for what it was created to do, and it will do whatever I commanded of it. I made the "few" adjustments the Holy Spirit instructed of me and since that first fifty-pound weight loss, I have had regular menstrual cycles.

He loves our bodies, even when we don't. He loves to watch when we defy the laws this world places against us. He loves to watch when we finally breakthrough. Because He already knows it will. He knew it would because He knows His work and He knows it very well.

See, this is what I choose to believe: When we come into the world with diseases and rare conditions, I don't believe God intends for us to use it as a crutch. When we live fulfilling, spontaneous lives, and then we're suddenly hit with cancer or osteoporosis, I don't believe God is saying your life is over. It is an attack of the enemy, and Yahweh is saying to you to overcome it. This does not mean you won't need protection. *"Put on the full armor of God,"* His word says, *"to stand against the devil's schemes"* (Ephesians 6:11, New International Version). This does not just apply to the physical body, but spirit, soul, and mind. Your body is a warrior's body, and as a warrior, there should never be a moment where you are not ready to war. Don't get caught slipping. Guard your body. Guard His temple. As you build up your mind, spirit, and soul with His word, your physical body will stand strong as well.

My body feels *more* than amazing when I'm obedient to His instructions, especially when it comes to my commitment to remain celibate. To many it seems crazy. It's an ancient practice that is usually disregarded because we feel that we need to answer our bodies' sexual desires. But truth is, our bodies are crying out to be listened to.

Back in 2009, when I lost my virginity, it was *not* my intention to remain celibate. By this, I thought I would be with the "man of my dreams" and we'd be exclusive with one another. I was ready to be a one woman's man *without* marriage and *without* it being acknowledged by God because I thought it was true love. In a sense, it was love but not the way I thought it'd be. So, when things went south with that "situation-ship" and Yahweh started to reveal to me my disobedience, I thought I had been lied to. I felt like I'd been fooled. But mind you, I'd been warned. Also, with this feeling of foolishness, it added to my list of why I was insignificant because my virginity was my weapon, my collateral if you will. I remember one guy friend even went as far as telling me the only reason he "pursued" me as hard as he did was because I was virgin, but since I'd "gave it up" I wasn't worthy of the chase. Those were not his exact words, but you get the picture. I was only worth something as long as my virginity was intact.

That did something to me. It wasn't long after that I'd made my mind up to remain celibate until marriage. But even as I made the decision, it was all for the wrong reasons. I made the decision to be worthy in the eyes of men. Not because I respected my body. Not because I didn't want another man to have to a piece of me. Not because I didn't want to glorify God with my body. Not because I wanted myself and others to understand that my body is His temple.

I now believe this is why singleness and celibacy were such a struggle at the beginning. I did not want to be single and I certainly did not want to feel lonely. Even though I was no longer a virgin, I found that many men still pursued when they learned that I'd only been *one* man, *one* time. So, for the first five years of my singleness at least, I struggled with longing for companionship, trying to force these relationships that God was just not budging on. It was either His way or no way.

Until it finally clicked: if these men were willing to chase me *for* my virginity or even for my lack of sexual experience, just how much was I really worth? And I don't mean sexually. Again, there was always some part of me aware of my connection to Christ and at this point in my life, I was well aware of His presence, even if I didn't always want to acknowledge Him. But in this, I couldn't separate myself from Christ because my body is His temple.

When you connect with another sexually, we are giving them a portion of us. And the more we're sexually involved, the stronger the bond grows. Not because of the act itself, but because of the feelings you have during the act. You become attached. Spiritually attached, whether good or bad. Then you're giving your all to this man or woman and giving nothing to the Father. Honoring this man or woman with your body, with *His* temple.

Are you getting the picture yet? Obviously, sex is meant to be enjoyable and meant for some form of connection. God created it, so He knows full well of its purpose. *But* our first commitment is to Christ. "We love because He first loved us" (1 John 4:19. New International Version). Why is this tremendously significant? We commit to Him so that He may guide us through circumstances, instruct us through trials, and protect us from the enemy's plans against His will. We commit to Him so that we may truly know what love is.

If I'd first consulted with God before allowing my emotions and feelings to rule my decisions, I would not have ignored the signs. I would not have fought to regain that portion of me I had given away. But because I'd given another His temple, I was punished. Not because He desired to throw His weight around. But because He loved me. Because I was and will always be His. Because the mandate was too strong to be overlooked.

Again, God is serious about His. His Son, Christ Jesus, lives in each of us. Galatians 2:20 says *"I have been crucified with Christ and I no longer live, but Christ lives in me, the life I now live in the body, I live by faith in the Son of God who loved me and gave himself for me"* (New International Version). You don't get to taint the body of Christ and think you won't have to answer to the Father. You cannot truly love another without growing closer to The Source of the love. A homeowner knows every part of their house, and they are willing to do whatever it takes to protect it. This is God. He'll put you out before He allows you to destroy it. His temple is His, not yours.

My celibacy and singleness journey is one of freedom; a journey that not only glorified God but intended to pull me closer to Him. In my singleness, I have been distraction free, allowing me to spend more time with Him, ridding the spirit of loneliness. It was not until I embraced my singleness and celibacy that I found comfort in God's Word, and *when* I understood my body was His - it was then that I found true peace and started to truly value who I am. And I'm perfect at this. But no man or his attention can place a bid on my value and win it. His only way to gain my body and my heart is to go through my Father Yahweh. And Yahweh knows me inside out, so the next man He places in my life will know exactly how to care for me, because he sought Him first. It all works out for your good if you just look at His greater picture, but what must we do? You should know the answer by now. It starts with *trust in Christ.*

Tashanda Mosley

6

WORSHIP!

I believe any man or woman can testify that we long for attention. To be desired. To be cared for, and to be appreciated and loved. Maybe the Father programmed it in our DNAs to long for that feeling - that warm, mushy feeling, that we'll spend our entire life searching for this perfect feeling.

In my opinion and from experience, worship gets you this feeling and so much more than you can ever expect. Worship is like a direct doorway to the Most High. The more you worship, the closer you grow in relationship to Him, the more you feel Him.

Worship surpasses loneliness. It cancels it completely out. Why? Because when Yahweh hears the cry of His children, He comes for them. He breaks down mountains. Worship takes your enemies by the necks and forces them to surrender and call out *their* sounds of defeat.

You worship those things that make you feel good. You worship those things that consume you. You worship what and/or who has been a "knight in shining armor" for you. You worship strongholds.

I have experienced it all. People and their ungodly behaviors and attention have consumed me. Things that make me feel like I'm floating on cloud 10; the men that have portrayed themselves as my knight in shining armor. The same men and desires that became heavy strongholds. Yes, I have, fortunately, gone through it all. And I say "fortunately" proudly, but humbly. Had I not experienced these things, I would not have known how much more powerful, how much more moving, and how much more loving God is for me. It took only a supernatural love and presence to loosen the chains and ropes these strongholds and sinful desires had on me.

I will never take the credit for these victories. I did not overcome alone. I did not come from the fire, purged, by myself. I went in alone, with no one or no one even knowing I was going. I went in with no one's support. The same strongholds, the same sexual and perverse desires that urged me on were nowhere to be found when I needed to climb my way out – or shall I say when He pushed me out. They were only present when they needed me and pushed me further down a slippery slope, not even considering my feelings, or the pain and the hurt. Or maybe they did consider it. Maybe they needed my soul to remain tainted and darkened because it would be the only way for me to keep allowing them back in. Maybe because they realized what God had called me to do long before I was aware, and to keep me off course, they needed me to stay down.

Because the devil knew that once I opened my mouth and started the howling worship to the Most High, He would come running. He would come down and he would rescue me. He would fill me with His empowering, overtaking, ground shaking strength to defeat my enemies that could once overpower me with just a few simple words... *"You can't do it..." "You are not enough..."*

But there was a mistake the devil made along the way. There was one thing that he *always* forgot to take heed of as he admired my decline. His plan was to make me feel more alone than before by excluding me, separating me from my favorite things and favorite people that made me accepted. If he could get my family and friends to the point where they could not understand me, if he could get me to no longer be encouraged by their presence, I would finally fall to my death. He could finally get me to take my own life.

But that was the biggest mistake that he could have ever made. When he thought he had gotten me alone, when thought he had me cornered, when he handed me the knife, he was so excited and wrapped up in my fall that he forgot about the Hovering.

See the devil often forgets that he was originally meant to worship too. And he thinks that if he can get us to rebel that he's winning and fighting against the will of God. But...he forgets that God will use us all, including him. Yes, God uses the devil. Every single time, he forgets that God will turn what he meant for bad into good. And he also forgets that Christ lives heavily and proudly in us.

All it takes is a faint cry, and the Spirit of Christ is alerted. And when we feel just a tiny bit of that Spirit, we cry out again. And He overpowers the darkness to get to us. And we feel Him consume us, then we yell out more to Him, *"Father, please... I need you."* Hearing this, He sends the devil and his demons into a trembling fear to find His child and He will not stop until we know that we are safe and covered.

Yep. He forgot that I was *never* alone. He forgot that God meant for me, meant for us, to be SET APART! Ha!

I'm here to tell you *right now* the devil never had you! He was only helping Yahweh. Father

Yahweh is getting ready to show you just how powerless that devil really is and just how powerful you really are. God is taking you back *right now*! The devil has had his fun for the last time on your behalf! That's some good news! That's enough for you to worship *Him right now* in the middle of reading this book! Get up right now and worship your Father!

Yes, I am a worshipper. I love to worship. I enjoy being as close to The Father as close as I can get, and worship gets me there. You can worship too. Worship is not meant to be boring. Worship is always meant to move—move you, move your circumstances, move Satan all the way back to hell where he came from.

Worship by Fasting

Isn't it amazing that something as "small" as what we eat and how much we eat is important to our Father? Doesn't it just mean so much to you that you mean so much to Him? It truly matters to Him how we treat our bodies.

I want to say this: all of this is from personal experiences; what worked for me. In no way will I force you to go by my rules just because it worked for me. But also let's be *clearer*: don't knock anything you have not tried for yourself. So, with that being said, working out did not lose the weight. Cutting back did not lose the weight. Starving myself definitely did not lose the weight. Fasting lost the weight. Not intermittent fasting, which is completely awesome by the way, but straight blown out fasting. I'm talking about liquid fasts and complete fasts; depriving yourself of pleasure foods type of fasts. Now before you say, "*Well you're starving yourself*," hear me out.

When I was full, when I had eaten those pleasure foods, I was in some way content with my situation, even as if it had not gone away. When I ate, I did not feel the desire to focus on the matter at hand and had the awful habit of pushing it away, up under a rug. When I had food on my stomach, I became sluggish, lacking motivation. Big time; and I found comfort in that. Food was my go-to. But a little over a year into my journey, I was re-introduced to fasting. The right way.

See, you can't fast properly with expectations of breaking bondages and generational curses without praying and connecting to Our Creator. And more than likely, the more you pray and connect to Yahweh, it becomes highly probable that He will ask you to fast. Because not only is it a sacrifice, but those strongholds and generational curses you're holding on to or choosing to ignore need to be broken for Him to use you fully. You are sacrificing something you love, something you've convinced yourself that you cannot live without to feed and strengthen your relationship with Him, fearing Him, trusting Him, submitting to Him. Not only that, He is teaching you obedience; and as we all know, obedience is better than sacrifice (1 Samuel 15:22).

When I began to fast again, I was at a point in my life where I'd gotten tired. Tired of failing. Tired of pushing forward. Tired of fighting. But I'd gotten so tired, I couldn't give up. At this point, I'd invested too much. I had expected too much to happen. It was also at this time, I had been at a standstill with my weight loss for about 9 months or so. I had maintained but I knew Our Father desired more of me, and when He wants more, He gets more. Not by force but because at some point the feeling to give Him more will be too strong to hold back. He'd already shown me through dreams how He desired me to look, and let me tell you, I looked good! At this point, He informed me fasting would be the only option. My only option for EVERYTHING I'd asked of Him, the entire list of my requests and promises. Fasting would be the only thing I could give Him. I tried to fight around it. Giving up social media. Cutting off men. No television for 21 days.

And don't get me wrong. It was definitely beneficial. There were breakthroughs. But it just made me more aware that it was not the fast Yahweh truly desired for me. And after saying, *"More of You, less of me"* and *"All of You, and none of me"* for so long, I could no longer ignore the fast that would BREAK ME THROUGH.

A 40 Day fast. While everyone at most churches took part in a twenty-one day fast to get the year started off right, Yahweh had started to prepare me to complete a 40 Day fast. Was I ready for it? At the time, I had no answer to that question. I was just tired of not being obedient. I was tired of being stuck in the same place, physically and spiritually. The fast was not specifically for my physical health. No, this fast was for my faith walk. It was meant for the dam to the breakthroughs that would break me all the way down — the breakthroughs that would move me out the way and *finally* allow Him to step in, in His rightful place in my life.

So going straight off of "dumb" faith, I took on the challenge of a 40 Day fast with another church member and spiritual sister, which was absolutely, completely unplanned. Neither of us knew at the time that we both were doing a 40 Day fast. It wasn't until we started to communicate on a day to day basis that we learned that the Holy Spirit had directed us to both do a 40 Day fast for different promises and visions but for the same reason: to be broken through. The fast actually started off intense and only got more intense. That's the thing about Yahweh: He starts out high. Being the Most High, He can't help but start out high and full of intensity. He's just that powerful. My fast consisted of fruits and vegetables, no processed foods, no dairy products, and water, water, water. Sometimes He directed me to do liquid fasts or a complete fast all together.

If I could truly describe the experience, this book would be completely burnt to smithereens: breaking bondages and chains, bounding up spirits, filling me with His fire, purging me, and taking me to a higher level of understanding and worship and praise. These words are nothing compared to the actual tasting and seeing of Him.

Worship in His Word

We are normally taught that reading is fundamental, right? That to be informed on how to successfully build that dollhouse or exercise bike, you need to carefully read the manual. Well, have you ever experienced a moment where this turned out to be false? I'm sure in some cases, God has shown you grace and worked things Himself, but for the most part if you don't read each instruction carefully, something is bound to go wrong and not work properly.

Well that's much like your new walk and the Holy Bible. As believers, especially new believers, we quite often wonder how to work out every situation we're placed in. And many times, when we result to our former life's habits, this makes the situation even stickier, right? Well, that's because when we were made new, He graced us with a clean slate. But also, because He cleansed us, He intends for nothing or no one, not even you to taint what He has purified. Father Yahweh loves us so, so much that He will allow you to go through the trenches before He allows you to disrespect your body, *His* temple.

But you don't have to go through what you went through in your former life, because you've been given a manual; The Manual. The Holy Bible is at your disposal, free for you to use at any moment, at any hour, at any situation, and I do literally mean, for *any* situation.

Yes, it works perfectly in your weight loss journey. It explores discipline. It talks gravely about fasting. It speaks heavily on loving yourself and others. It's built around faith. It heals you out of that destructive relationship. It prepares you for ministry. I can give you scripture after scripture that has pushed me and is pushing me through my journey. *"Worship the Lord your God, and his blessing will be on your food and water, I will take away sickness from among you, and none will miscarry or be barren in your land; I will give you a full life span* (Exodus 23:25-26, NIV). *"Do not conform to the pattern of this world, but be transformed by the renewing of your mind, then you will be able to test and approve what God's will is—his good, pleasing, and perfect will"* (Romans 12:2, NIV). *"You were bought with a price, therefore honor God with your bodies"* (1 Corinthians 6:20). And finally, Isaiah 40:29-31, which is what *Walking in Newness* was created on, *"He gives strength to the weary and increases the power of the weak, even youths grown tired and weary, and young men stumble and fall; but those who hope in the Lord will renew their strength; they will soar on wings like eagles; they will run and not grow weary, they will walk and not be faint,"* (NIV).

Honey, there's so much more where that comes from. Those examples are just a scratch on the surface. My goal is not to write out the Bible for you; it's to push you go check it out for yourself. His Word holds your answer, and it's waiting to be discovered by you. I'm willing to bet you have asked God the same question over and over again, and you've passed up your Bible as an option, substituting your best friend instead. We make the excuse that the Bible is too boring and too much to read. Well how would you feel if God says you're too disobedient and disregards you when you finally turn to Him when life gets too much to handle alone? It wouldn't feel so good?

To know Him is love Him. But you can't know Him if you don't search His word. Read His word. Test His word. Then believe Him.

Worship in Music

Close family and friends know that I am a music lover. I love it all. *NSYNC and Christina Aguilera were my favorite artists. I was in a so-called girl band from middle school to high school. The name changed a lot, but the one I remember is Lil' Luxuries. I think we were all determined to be superstars, so we can marry members of a boy band. A girl can dream right?

Music was always a primary outlet when people let me down or when my plans didn't go as I'd hoped - and nothing has changed to this day. I just found a different type of music as an outlet. Worship music. See how God will you use anything! Because it's His anyway! You cannot get away from Him that easy.

Yes, I found music in worship. No, I cannot sing. But honey, when I get in the spirit, don't think I won't try whatever gets me connected to Him. I think next to exercising, music is probably my favorite form of worship. You should see my playlists!

Music and lyrics are influencing. Together, they are enticing and inspiring, and God created them. Imagine what happens when you worship God with music and words. Yes, power is the word. In prayer, I use music. In the gym, I use music. As I write, I use music. As I'm cleaning, I use music. When I'm sleeping, I use music. At all hours, my goal is to worship Yahweh.

Why is worship important in your newness? Because Christ is your newness, and our number one goal is to worship Him. My pastor always says, *"Our job is to blow God up!"* I know. Sometimes we get distracted. Life in this world can be overbearing. But make a conscious effort to get in His presence because that's where He provides your escape, your tactics, your assignments, and your rest. It's never boring in Yahweh's presence. In His presence, you see the fighting. You see the fire. You see His glory.

There's a shaking there. Your newness is in the worship!

7

That Little Boy or That Little Girl

Now finally, to you. You didn't think I'd forgotten about you, did you? I could never. I was once "there" where you think you are.

First things first: You are not your circumstances. You are not defined by your circumstances. Do not be moved by your circumstances. They are only there for one of two reasons: to distract you or to motivate you. But God does not place you in circumstances to make you feel good. He places you there to change you—not changed by you but by Him. However, your circumstances are not meant to be permanent. Let go of that lie right now, IN THE MIGHTY NAME OF JESUS!

I know you've always felt like you were nothing. Like you are less than the bottoms of shoes walking through garbage. They told you that you're too fat. They told you that you weren't handsome enough. That told you can't defeat poverty. They put you in a bubble and made you believe that you were limited to that teeny tiny bubble. Let go of that lie right now, IN THE MIGHTY NAME OF JESUS!

You've wanted to give up. You've wanted to take your own life. You've believed that your existence was insignificant. Depression has consumed you. Worldly acceptance has tainted you. Fear has hindered you. Get rid of this lie, IN THE MIGHTY NAME OF JESUS!

HE said you are created in His image and that you have dominion over the earth (Genesis 1:26-27). HE said you are more than a conqueror through Christ Jesus who loved us (Romans 8:37). HE said that his grace is sufficient for you, and that His power is made perfect in your weakness (2 Corinthians 12:9). You are fearfully and wonderfully made (Psalm 139:14). HE SAID. HE SAID this! HE cannot lie!

Let go of that abusive relationship! Let go of that degrading job! Let go of the fear of falling! Let go of what you like and go after Him who loves you! He will meet you right where you are, even if that's right in the devil's hands!

You are more than enough! You are not a mistake. You have a for sure purpose! You have a duty and a right to protect your promises and your inheritance! Get out of the lie and declare on this day that you were created by a perfect God and that the enemy is defeated IN THE MIGHTY NAME OF JESUS! Feeling sorry for yourself does not move mountains! Decrees shatter mountains! Fighting shatters mountains! Faith shatters mountains! Freedom shatters mountains!

Daniel 1:8-21

But Daniel resolved not to defile himself with the royal food and wine, and he asked the chief official for permission not to defile himself this way. Now God had caused the official to show favor and compassion to Daniel, but the official told Daniel, "I am afraid of my lord the king, who has assigned your food and drink. Why should he see you looking worse than the other young men your age? The king would then have my head because of you."Daniel then said to the guard whom the chief official had appointed over Daniel, Hananiah, Mishael and Azariah. "Please test your servants for ten days: Give us nothing but vegetables to eat and water to drink. Then compare our appearance with that of the young men who eat the royal food, and treat your servants in accordance with what you see." So he agreed to this and tested them for ten days. At the end of the ten days they looked healthier and better nourished than any of the young men who ate the royal food. So the guard took away their choice food and the wine they were to drink and gave them vegetables instead. To these four young men God gave knowledge and understanding of all kinds of literature and learning. And Daniel could understand visions and dreams of all kinds. At the end of the time set by the king to bring them into his service, the chief official presented them to Nebuchadnezzar. The king talked with them, and he found none equal to Daniel, Hananiah, Mishael and Azariah; so they entered the king's service. In every matter of wisdom and understanding about which the king questioned them, he found them ten times better than all the magicians and enchanters in his whole kingdom. And Daniel remained there until the first year of King Cyrus.

Believe the hype: The food you eat is REALLY 80% (90% if you ask me) of your weight loss, or weight gain; however you choose to look at it - IT REALLY MATTERS. Between November 2017 and February 2018, I lost at least 40 lbs, and I might've worked out seven times. Maybe. Now I truly encourage an active lifestyle. That 20% is necessary. I would not take it back for the world. I will always support exercising. But exercising will mean absolutely nothing if the foods you eat are not aligned with it. You cannot work out 5 times a week and eat greasy, fried foods afterwards and expect real results.

Why less meat (or no meat) and no dairy is better (FOR ME!):

I want to constantly stress that my goal is to maintain a healthy lifestyle without meat and dairy. It's not perfected but it's definitely a daily habit. It works for me. THIS DOES NOT HAVE TO AN OPTION FOR YOU. My body feels better, and it thanks me every day for it. I sleep better. I'm more alert. It just works for me. When I did the 40 Day fast, it was the first thing my inner spirit told me to get rid of. Started off a bit rough, but as time progressed, I found I didn't desire it as much. So, here's a list of recommended foods to try.

100% Juice (NO ADDED SUGARS)

Olive Oil

Coconut Oil

Avocado Oil

Sea Salt

Black Pepper

Bell Peppers (all colors)

Sweet Potatoes

Spinach

Romaine

Celery

Parsley

Cilantro

Ginger

Avocados (high in fat)

Potatoes (in moderation for low starch intake)

Cauliflower

Carrots

Squash

Zucchini

Mushrooms

Broccoli

Tomatoes (fresh or canned w/ less preservatives and chemicals as possible)

Legumes (dry or canned w/ less preservatives and chemicals as possible)

Broth (better homemade to control sodium intake)

Collard greens (fresh)

Kale greens (fresh)

Cabbages

Almond Milk

Coconut Milk

Brown Rice

Chickpeas

Quinoa

Oatmeal

Flax seeds

Chia seeds

Sesame seeds

Sunflower seeds

Tofu

Strawberries

Bananas (eat in moderation for low sugar intake)

Oranges (eat in moderation for low sugar intake)

Blueberries

Raspberries

Blackberries

Plums

Watermelon

Cherries

Grapes

Nectarines

Cranberries

Lemons

Limes

Pineapples (fresh recommended, canned contains high amounts of sugar)

Peaches (fresh recommended)

Kiwi

Apples

Mangoes

Raw/Organic Honey

Coconut sugar

Agave

Blue Corn tortillas chips

Whole wheat tortillas

Multigrain loaf bread
(in moderation)

Corn (fresh and
canned)

Green beans

Sweet Peas

Hummus

Apple Cider Vinegar

Salmon (fresh or
frozen)

Turkey (fresh and
frozen)

Chicken

Rice flour

Oat flour

Chickpea flour

Tapioca flour

All-Purpose flour**

All natural peanut
butter (no extra
chemicals and sugars)

EAT AS MUCH **RAW FRUITS AND VEGETABLES AS POSSIBLE**

Cabbage Soup

Ingredients:
1/2 head of cabbage, chopped

1 cup celery, diced

1 cup white or yellow onion, diced

1 cup carrots, diced

1 green bell pepper, diced

2-3 cloves garlic, minced

4 cups vegetable/chicken broth

14 oz can basil, oregano, garlic diced tomatoes

1 teaspoon oregano

1 teaspoon basil

1/2 teaspoon red pepper flakes

Few shakes of black pepper

1/2 teaspoon salt (optional)

Heat 2 tablespoons of olive oil in a large pot over medium heat. Add celery, onions, bell peppers, and carrots. Sauté until slightly tender. Stir in garlic. Pour in chicken broth. Stir in tomatoes and cabbage. Bring to a boil and then reduce heat. Cook until cabbage is tender. Stir in oregano, basil, red pepper flakes, black pepper and salt (if using). Taste broth and adjust seasoning if needed.

Vegetarian BBQ Burrito Bowl

Ingredients:

1 Avocado

1 cup BBQ sauce

1 batch Black beans

2 cups Rice

1 Salt

2 tsp Cumin

Tortilla chips

Cook rice according to directions on package. Heat the black beans as well before taking all other ingredients, including rice and mix up together. Season to liking.

Turkey Taco Lettuce Wraps

Ingredients:

1 Tbsp olive oil

3/4 cup chopped yellow onion

1 lb 95% lean ground turkey

2 cloves garlic

Salt and freshly ground black pepper

1 Tbsp chili powder

1 tsp ground cumin

1/2 tsp paprika

1/2 cup tomato sauce

1/2 cup low-sodium chicken broth

Iceberg or Romaine lettuce leaves, doubled up, for serving

Heat olive oil in a non-stick skillet over medium-high heat. Add onion and sauté 2 minutes. Add turkey and garlic, then season with salt and pepper; cook, tossing and breaking up turkey occasionally, until cooked thoroughly, about 5 minutes. Add chili powder, cumin, paprika, tomato sauce and chicken broth. Reduce to a simmer and cook about 5 minutes until sauce has reduced. Serve mixture over lettuce leaves with desired toppings.

Spicy Black Bean Burger

Ingredients:

1 15 oz. can Black beans

1 Carrot, medium-sized

1/2 cup Cilantro, fresh

1/2 cup Corn

1/2 tsp Garlic

1/2 Jalapeno

1 Red bell pepper

1/3 Red onion

1/2 cups Oats

1/4 tsp Black pepper

1/2 tsp Chili powder

2 tbsp Nutritional yeast

1/2 tsp Paprika

3/4 tsp Sea salt

1 tsp Cumin, ground

2 tbsp Flaxseed, ground

1/4 cup Breadcrumbs (in my opinion, this is not needed)

1 whole wheat Burger buns (optional)

1/3 cup of water

On the stovetop, heat a pan over medium-high heat. Add the water (or oil, if not oil-free) and sauté the onion, jalapeño and garlic until soft, about 4-5 minutes. Turn off heat and set aside.

In a food processor, blend up the oats to make a flour. Add in the breadcrumbs, ground flax, nutritional yeast, cumin, sea salt, chili powder, paprika and black pepper. Blend until well combined and transfer this dry mixture to a large bowl. Into the food processor, add the red bell pepper, carrot and cilantro. Blend/pulse until finely shredded (don't overdo it or the veggies will get too watery). Transfer to the large bowl with the dry mixture. Into the food processor add the black beans and blend until mashed, with a few black beans still intact, for texture. Transfer to the large bowl. Add in the corn and the sautéed onion mixture. Mix together with your hands. It is the best way! Then form into 5 patties. Lay them flat on a plate and cover with plastic wrap. Refrigerate for 30 minutes to set. This step is crucial! Remove from refrigerator and heat up the same pan on medium heat. Spray with nonstick spray and cook each patty until golden/browned, about 4 minutes on each side. Serve on a bun or over a salad with all the toppings

Tomato Basil Soup

Ingredients:

Canned tomatoes (whole or stewed)
Fresh tomatoes

Garlic cloves

1-2 Potatoes

Onions

Red bell peppers

Chicken/Vegetable broth

Basil (fresh or dried)

With tomato soup, you can go the quick route and pour canned tomatoes in a pot and simmer them for 15-20 minutes until they're soft. However, going that extra step and roasting tomatoes along with whole (smashed) garlic cloves on a sheet pan until they're soft and sweetened naturally with their own juices, develops a natural flavor incomparable to canned soup. I use a humble potato to thicken this soup. Of course, you can leave them out if you wish, but they add a thick and creamy texture and compliment the tomato flavor that I suggest leaving it in. Frying them while your tomatoes are roasting, with diced onion and red bell peppers, until the onion is transparent, and the potatoes are beginning to crisp up adds even more flavor into this soup. Then pour in your broth/stock and simmer the potatoes until they're soft. Add the tomatoes once they're done; add the basil; blitz with a stick blender, and voila! SOUP!

Baked Salmon

Ingredients:

Fresh or frozen salmon

1 lemon

Lemon pepper seasoning

Dried oregano

Cilantro

Sea salt

Black pepper

Olive oil or coconut oil

Salmon can be thawed or frozen. Cover salmon with oil. Sprinkle on seasoning, careful not to over-season. Cut up cilantro and sprinkle over top. Cut up lemon and lay over salmon. Put in 350-degree preheated oven for 15-20 minutes if salmon is thawed, 20-30 minutes if salmon is frozen.

***Can eat with spinach salad

Spinach Salad

Ingredients:

2 cups of Spinach leaves

1 Tomato or 1 cup of cherry tomatoes

1 cucumber

Sunflower seeds (optional)

Avocado Dressing for Salad (can store in refrigerator for up to one week)

Ingredients:

1 Avocado

Olive oil

Lemon juice

Sea Salt

Black pepper

Use blender to combine all ingredients. If you don't have blender, use a whisk. Make sure you blend thoroughly.

Vegetable Soup

Ingredients:

Frozen vegetables

*Corn

*Sweet Peas

*Green beans

*Carrots

Potatoes

Canned tomatoes

Lemon Pepper

Italian seasoning

Black Pepper

Paprika

Parsley (dried or fresh)

Salsa (medium heat) or canned tomato paste

Vegetable broth

Boil potatoes until soft but not breaking apart. Drain. Pour in all tomatoes and tomato paste or salsa, along with seasonings. Pour in vegetable broth. Simmer for 15-20 minutes or until tomatoes have softened and browned down. Mix in the vegetables. Cook until vegetables are soft or to your liking

Infused Water

Water (I find distilled water is better)

Fresh or frozen fruit (fresh fruit works better)

Stevia drops (optional)

(Let water set at least one hour. Throw away fruit after 24 hours)

Infused Water Detox

Cucumbers

Mint

Lemons

Curry Chick Pea Spinach and Tomato Stew

Ingredients:

Chickpeas (canned)

Lentils (canned or dry)

Tomatoes (diced, stewed)

Spinach (1/2 cup)

Kale (1/2 cup)

Onion (half)

Garlic (1 clove)

Olive oil (or coconut oil)

Vegetable stock (can use chicken stock)

Italian seasoning

Parsley

Paprika

Sea salt

Lemon Pepper seasoning

Chili powder

Turmeric

Quinoa (1/4 cup)

Corn starch (for thickening)

Heat oil in pan. Finely chop onions and garlic. Place in heated oil and brown. Drained chickpeas, lentils, and tomatoes. Pour in 1/2 cup of stock. Let it come to a simmer, then pour in canned tomatoes. Add seasoning for taste (You do not have to use all the seasonings I used. Customize however you'd like). Let it come to a simmer again and let it cook for about 15 minutes. Rinse and pour in quinoa. Stir stew, then cover. You'll mix the corn starch with a little water, but DO NOT POUR IN UNTIL quinoa is cooked. The quinoa will also act as a thickener, so you may not even need the corn starch. After the quinoa is cooked and you desire a thicker consistency, pour in corn starch mix at that point. If you'd like a thinner stew, pour in more vegetable stock or water to control sodium input. Allow stew to thicken for another minute or two. Then put it washed spinach and kale leaves. Stir in until wilted down and turn off stove.

BBQ Cauliflower Wings

Ingredients:

Head of cauliflower

Wild Thymes Whistlin' Dixie Barbecue Sauce (any vegan will do. Just make sure it's natural and healthy)

Olive oil/Coconut oil

Flour (any flour from the recommended list will do)

Sea salt

Black pepper

Oregano

Chili powder

Lemon pepper seasoning

Water

Break cauliflower into desired wing pieces. Wash thoroughly. In a bowl, mix flour with seasonings. Pour in water until mixture is a semi-thin consistency. Put in cauliflower. Cover completely. Now you have two options: bake or fry. This is one of the recipes where frying would be okay. However, I recommend trying both methods. For baking, cover non-stick pan with a thin coat of oil or you can use parchment paper. Place cauliflower wings on pan and paper. Put in preheated 350-degree oven. Bake for 35 minutes. Half way through, flip cauliflower over. Cook until brown. Carefully place wings in sauce. Cover entirely. Put wings back on baking sheets. Place back in oven and bake for another 15 minutes or until brown.

These are just a few suggestions that I think you should try out because they are absolutely awesome. But feel free to go to Pinterest and find more recipe options.

I truly, truly hope this helps. If just one person finds something out of this, and applies it to their everyday life, you'll find positive results. I'm still very new to this and I think I will always be in constant learning mode as it took me 29 years to realize my body was crying out for help. I'm learning something new about my body every day. And I can only give credit to God for bringing me to this point. I pray each of you find something worthwhile and we can all grow together as we learn to listen to our bodies and take better care of them.

NOTES:

You may notice there are some foods that I have not included on either list. That's because this is a suggested list. These are the foods I ate to help with my weight loss journey. For instance, bread would probably be a no-go for me. Most breads are not helpful on my journey. Breads tended to make me full, too full. So full, I could not function after 30 minutes or so. I felt way too heavy. If I do have breads, it'll be tortillas, whole wheat or multi-grain or unleavened breads.

Same thing with meats. After I completed a 40 Day fast with no meats - when I did start to consume meats again, my body reacted differently, usually having cramps, or indigestion, and extreme heaviness. So, I am going to strongly recommend and encourage you to go a day without meat. Start off with just one day a week. I'm willing to bet you've done it before. You just weren't conscious of it. With you making a conscious effort, it will seem tougher. However, with practice and research (and PRAYER), you'll be able to find foods that resemble the texture of meats, will be as filling as meat, and carry just as much protein as meat, if not much more!

Sugars... I know I'm going to step on some toes with this one. But let's face it: Sugars are NOT our friend! I don't care how good it is at the time. It's like a bad ex we can't get rid of: always whispering sweet NOTHINGS to us. We have to let the processed sugars go. I recommend stevia and honey (in moderation). But try going a week without sugar, and watch the weight fall off. I've seen what no sugars and no starches do. Not for me but for others. My pastor and wife removed sugars and starches from their diet, just sugars and starches, and their body was transformed before the congregation's very eyes. If you have plenty of fruit, they'll suffice and satisfy those sugar cravings.

Flours: In my experience with flour since my weight loss, it hasn't harmed me much unless it was eating fried foods excessively. I don't use self-rising flour. I believe flours can be used but in moderation and I don't say that lightly. Don't include flour as a part of your daily diet. A little in a recipe every now and then is fine. But the goal is to get the weight off and because flour is starchy, it has a lot of carbohydrates. I don't count carbs or calories, but I do use common senses. Now if you intend to have a high intense workout regime, this may work out great for you as carbohydrates are supposed to give you energy. You know what works for your body and what doesn't.

Diet drinks are not healthy! Period. They usually contain processed sugars or artificial sugars, which mean one thing: chemicals. This doesn't include the chemicals used to make the drinks itself. To be honest, while I included juice and tea, for weight loss, your best choice is always going to be water. Water, water, water. I cannot stress this enough. Free of chemicals and it flushes your body out. If you'd like a little taste, try infused water. If you *have* to have a little sugar, use stevia with your water.

Workout Regime

Note: It's important to remember that this workout regime as well as the recommended food list is what worked for ME. Many have asked and I'm simply giving instructions on how I've lost weight thus far. As time progresses, I'm certain your regime will change as your body adapts to your workout; you must keep your body in constant shock to continue weight loss. However, in my opinion, you don't have to be drastic with workout exercises to lose weight effectively. But there should be a constant effort and you should be open to new challenges.

Walking: Very simple but don't underestimate its effectiveness. Walking works the entire body and is a form of cardio.

Jogging: I recommend jogging as you walk. Again, it shocks the body by increasing your heart rate, as well helps to increase your endurance.

Running: I know for some, running is a challenge, especially for my fellow heavy bodies. But the jogging helps you work your way up to running. And again, IT'S CARDIO: it works the heart, burns fat, and boosts your metabolism, which all promotes and triggers weight loss.

Boxing: More of a hobby than anything for me. But boxing works the arms and it works your core. Start off boxing for two minutes. Break for 1 minute. Repeat 3x

Triceps dips: 3 sets of 15 reps

Crunches: 3 sets of 10 reps

Sumo squats: 2 sets of 10 reps

Jump squats: 2 sets of 10 reps

Russian twists: 2 sets of 15

Mountain climbers: 2 sets of 10 reps

Skaters: 2 sets of 15 reps

High Knee Lifts: 30 seconds, 3 sets reps

Planks: 30/60 seconds, 2 sets (I like the full plank and elbow plank) reps

Of course, the gym offers great equipment to help with weight loss, such as:

Stair Climber

Elliptical

Cable Biceps Bar

Rowing Machine

Yoga

Zumba

Again, these are literally just a FEW. Of course, you're allowed to do any exercise you feel fit to do. Have fun with it. Do some research and find exercises you'd like to try. As a heavier person, sometimes we have to find moderation versions until our body will allow it. Also, as a heavier person, you tend to lose weight quicker in the beginning because you're utilizing your own body weight, if you're consistent and faithful to the journey. Just always keep in mind to challenge yourself. Weight loss doesn't come by being comfortable. It's absolutely uncomfortable but the rewarding feeling you have masks it all!

FASTING! I know I covered it in the book, but if you need to, go back and read it again. Fasting is extremely important! Whether it's intermittent fasting, partial fasting, complete fasting, or liquid fasting, it is absolutely great for the body - physically but more importantly spiritually. Fasting causes you to sacrifice food for time with the Father. When we eat, we're satisfied. We're too full to function, too full to be alert. When we're fasting, our senses are extremely sensitive. As humans, we don't like discomfort. But in fasting, you face a lot of discomfort. But that discomfort helps you gain spiritual clarity. It also intensifies intimacy with Yahweh, pieces of your flesh will die, allowing the manifestation of the Holy Spirit to occur more. Honestly speaking, if I had not fast when instructed, I would not have lost the weight that I have. I will tell anyone, for me, this is more of a spiritual journey than weight loss journey. God knew how unhappy I was with being overweight and the emotions and health issues that came with it. He developed the perfect regimen to lose it. But it required my attention to be focused on Him. In doing so, I've lost over 100lbs thus far. Fasting works! It doesn't seem ideal but if you've tried everything else and nothing has worked, what will it hurt to try this? I'm just saying.

Once again, all of these are JUST recommendations. You may read this and feel like it won't work for you and that's completely fine. But don't give up on life. Don't just exist. *Live*.

To My Family: My Apologies

I know these past couple of years have been a bit...
different with me. I won't say "tough" because for
me "amazing", "marvelous", or "life-altering" would
be the words I would use. But for many of you, my
transformation came suddenly and unintentionally
inconspicuous. So inconspicuous, many of you lost
understanding of who I was. Relationships changed,
and I may have offended a few of you. I pushed
myself away from my family, as I thought you all
just didn't understand. Too many times, I was told
to tone down my passion for words and love for
God, by a few of you all. So, when the battle of
depression, low self-esteem, and suicidal thoughts
took a major toll several years ago, my first mind
was to NOT speak to any of you about it. And I
admit: there were a few of you asking about me. But
by this time, I was too self-conscious of what you'd
think of me. For so long, I'd been forced to hush
about my problems and listen to others. For so long,
I forgot that I was allowed to be included in "others"

too. For so long, the enemy fooled me into thinking that I was not important. For so long, I thought some of you were my enemy. And that truly hurt. I separated myself from you all. For this, I apologize.

I apologize for all the times I didn't contact you because of pride. I apologize for making you feel like you couldn't be included in my newness. I apologize for sometimes not seeming normal. I apologize for withholding from you. I apologize for not loving you the way Christ loves us. I apologize for failing you as a daughter, sister, cousin, niece, auntie, godmother, or friend.

But the beautiful thing about walking in newness is I don't have to make those same mistakes again. I can forgive. I can include as many of you as I want; and I want each and every one of you with me, ALL UP IN MY NEWNESS!

I love you!

Tashanda Mosley

About the Author

Tashanda was born and raised in the Mississippi Delta. She's a proud graduate of Mississippi University for Women and Liberty University, where she received her Master's Degree in Human Services Counseling in Marriage and Family. Nine years celibate and eight years single, she believes that every male and every female, young and old, should make a conscious effort to worship and honor God with their bodies. As an obesity survivor, by making her relationship with Christ a priority, she has been able to maintain a healthy, active lifestyle and aims profusely to impact and educate her community on healthy living and sustaining an unassailable relationship with God.

Walking in Newness is built on the scripture Isaiah 40:29-31, *"He gives strength to the weary and increases the power of the weak. Even youths grow tired and weary, and young men stumble and fall, but those who hope in the Lord will renew their strength, they will soar on wings like eagles; they will run and not grow weary, they will walk and not be faint."*